Overcoming Occupational Burnout

A Practical Guide for Getting Your Life Back

Matthew Spencer Flynn

Copyright © 2020 Matthew Spencer Flynn

All Rights Reserved

ISBN: 9798696139449

Table of Contents

Introduction

Once, not so long ago, you thought you'd found your dream job. You were so excited about the interview and couldn't wait to get started. Every small success was a reason to celebrate; you were always focused and motivated even for long hours at work. You thought it must be your life's purpose. You considered yourself blessed to have this dream job.

But now, things are significantly different. You hate Mondays; all you want in the morning is to stay in bed, hide under the covers, and never have to show up at that office again. It's hard to find motivation for even minor tasks, let alone staying focused. You find yourself procrastinating and having angry outbursts at your colleagues and loved ones outside the workplace. It's almost impossible to concentrate. You don't feel skilled anymore. You can't even feel excitement or happiness at any achievement. You don't feel able to accomplish anything.

Might it be time to change careers? But you invested so much time and effort into building it. It used to be your dream job, for god's sake! You have no energy for finishing simple tasks, let alone contemplate a career change. Moreover, even if you could, you are pretty sure that it wouldn't make things any better. Your whole life is suffering. It might seem like you have put too much of yourself into work, that your job swallowed everything. You are so consumed that you have no energy for your loved ones and your life outside the workplace is neglected.

If any of this sounds like you, you might be suffering from occupational burnout.

What Is Occupational Burnout?

Do you know that feeling when you do something so much that you get sick of it? Well, that's the shortest explanation of occupational burnout.

Work burnout, as it's also known, is a condition characterized by exhaustion. It might be physical, emotional, intellectual, or all of them together. One feels drained and empty, with no energy or will for work. It occurs due to prolonged work-related stress and affects one's life in many ways.

Burnout is not an official medical diagnosis, but according to some experts, there are other conditions behind burnout, such as depression. Many people who experience burnout don't even believe that their job is the main cause.

Official diagnosis or not, occupational burnout can majorly affect your physical and mental health. That's why it is important to recognize if you're experiencing occupational burnout and then consider how to recover from it.

How to Tell If You're Suffering from Burnout

Do any of the following sound familiar?

- You feel a constant lack of energy.
- Your sleeping habits have changed. You sleep the whole day, or have trouble falling or staying asleep.
- You have to force yourself to go to work and it's tough for you to get started.
- You've become impatient and irritable with people around you, especially at work—co-workers, clients, and customers.
- You've become critical and cynical about work and people at work.
- You lack the energy to be as productive as you need to.
- It's hard for you to concentrate and stay focused.
- You don't care about your achievements anymore; they no longer bring you joy.
- You have no more illusions or passion for your job.
- You're are using food to feel better.
- You're using alcohol or drugs to feel better or to not think about what's bothering you.
- You suffer from headaches.

- You experience unexplained stomach or intestinal problems, or other random pain.

If any of the above refers to you, you might be experiencing job burnout. First, you need to see a doctor or a mental health provider to rule out other possible causes. If there's no other diagnosis or condition provoking it, chances are your job is the element out of balance.

Although it's not an official medical diagnosis, that doesn't mean it's not dangerous. Occupational burnout is not something you should have to live with. That sense of emptiness and exhaustion is not normal. There are many things that can help you recover and bring back your energy and life satisfaction.

Possible Causes and Risk Factors

Before we start searching for the solutions to our problems, most of us like to know what causes them in the first place. And it makes sense: if you know the source of your troubles, you can eliminate it or at least minimize its impact.

So what could be the cause of occupational burnout?

A LOT of constant stress

Job burnout is not the same as stress from work. Stress is a normal part of our daily lives and careers, and it won't cause damage if it's managed well. But if you are constantly exposed to high levels of stress and do nothing about mitigating it, it will lead to burnout.

Work-life imbalance

If your job consumes so much of your energy that you don't have time for family, friends, and other things that make your personal life fulfilling, you'll burn out quickly.

Lack of social connections and support

Social isolation at work and in your personal life is a risk factor for many kinds of mental health issues.

Job burnout is not an exception. If you feel isolated, you'll experience higher levels of stress and be more prone to burnout.

Monotony or chaos

When a job is chaotic or monotonous, you need more energy to stay focused. This drains you, creating higher levels of stress leading to adrenal fatigue and occupational burnout.

Dysfunctional personal relationships in the workplace

If you feel undermined by colleagues, unappreciated by your boss, or you work with an office bully or other kind of toxic co-worker, it won't be enough to love your job. We all need to feel accepted and connected, and our workplace is not an exception. If you work with people and don't feel good in their company, it drains your energy and sets you on the path to burnout.

Unclear expectations

If you are not clear about what your duty is, what level of authority you have, and what others expect from you, you can't feel comfortable. It can be particularly stressful trying to meet someone else's expectations when you don't even know what they are. If you lack feedback, you can't know if you are on the right path, which makes the stress worse.

<u>Lack of control</u>

If you have no influence on decisions that affect your job, such as workload, schedule, and assignments, or you don't have enough resources to complete the job, you might feel powerless and stressed. This feeling of not being in control of things that affect your life leads to burnout, too.

Almost anyone can experience occupational burnout at some point in life. However, there are some factors that could make you more likely to experience it. Here are some of them:

- Your job is to help people. Employees in the service professions, such as the health care sector, are more prone to burnout.
- You work A LOT. High workload, a busy schedule, and overtime hours are risk factors for job burnout.
- You identify with your work. If you do this and neglect your personal life, it creates an imbalance, which leads to burnout.
- You are doing too much on your own. If you try to do everything by yourself, it's time to learn how to delegate. Also, if you don't set

healthy boundaries and try to be there for everyone, you are at high risk.

- You have too little impact and control over your work. Someone else is in charge of your schedule, workload, and assignments.
- You find your job to be dull and monotonous.
- You feel lonely and isolated at your workplace or in your personal in life.

What If You Do Nothing About It?

Occupational burnout is not an illness, it's a condition. It's not a medical diagnosis, but that doesn't mean it can't lead to some serious health and mental issues. You might think it's not your job that causes you to feel like this. Or you think you are just tired, you need a rest, some time away from work, and everything will fall back into place.

There is some truth in this. It's not only your job that causes the problem; you really need rest and some time away from your duties. But this is not all. A vacation, even a terrific one, won't fix things completely. Job burnout didn't happen overnight. So it's not realistic to expect it to disappear just like that. Recovery will take time and effort.

If you don't address or try to ignore job burnout, the only thing you can expect is for it to get worse and cause additional problems.

This might include:

- More and more stress
- Chronic fatigue
- Sleeping problems, insomnia
- Sadness and depression
- Anxiety and panic

- Irritability, outbursts of anger, and problems controlling your rage
- Alcohol abuse
- Drug use
- High blood pressure
- Heart disease
- Type 2 diabetes
- Low immune system and vulnerability to illnesses
- Problems in personal interactions
- Lower quality of life in general

These are just some of the consequences if occupational burnout goes unaddressed and is not confronted. Obviously, it's a serious condition that requires you to take it seriously and do whatever is in your power to solve it. Last but not least, you have only one life. Do you really want to spend it tired, grumpy, cynical, and desperate?

How to Recover

1.   Recognize the problem

As always, recognition and becoming aware of the problem is the first step towards solving it. You need to be honest with yourself and admit how you feel. It's not a sign of weakness to admit that you are exhausted, no longer happy, and that something should change.

Make a doctor's appointment to check your overall health. Your physician will want to rule out any other possible causes of your issues. If there's nothing else that is provoking these feelings and if anything or everything from the list above refers to you, it's probably occupational burnout.

There are different kinds of burnout: general, emotional, and occupational. They all have a lot in common, but there are also specific differences among them. Job burnout doesn't necessarily mean that you hate your job or need to change your career, it just means that something about your job is the main cause of high stress, leading to burnout. So admit how you really feel about your job and think about what's affecting you. Is it too little time for your personal life, the sense that you lack control, work with a bully, or something else?

Once you realize that your condition is occupational burnout, it's time to start taking steps towards overcoming it.

2.   Press pause

It would be naive to think that sleeping longer a night or two or going on vacation will solve the problem, but it would be worthwhile to take a pause. It might be a few days off, a vacation, or any kind of extra time free from work. Maybe you can't cancel all of your duties, but try to adjust your schedule and free it from any non-necessary tasks. Ask your boss, employer, or clients for patience; postpone what can wait. Make yourself and your recovery a priority and reserve enough time for it.

It's time to do what you usually don't—to cancel or postpone certain tasks and duties in order to rest and pay attention to your private life instead. Delegate what you can; the rest can wait. You'll be surprised to realize that your career will not be over if you take a break.

3.   Reach out for help

It's not a sign of weakness to reach out for help when you need it. Burnout is one of those cases. You need to talk to someone. It can be a friend, a trusted family member, or a professional. You can choose   among   life-coaches,   therapists, psychologists. But the crucial thing is to talk to someone. Even if your friend or a family member doesn't have a solution to your issue, you'll feel lighter and you'll have a clearer picture of what's going on. If you decide for a coach or a therapist, they will probably lead you to some constructive solutions for your situation. Also, this book is here to help you go through this phase as painlessly as possible and find solutions on your own.

It's much easier to handle things when you know you are not alone. Don't hesitate to connect with people around you, even if you don't want to talk about what's bothering you. Remember that social isolation is one of the risk factors for developing burnout, but also one of the factors that interfere with recovery.

4.   Find the causes of the problem

The roots of occupational burnout are more or less the same—too much work, too little rest, and insufficient joy. However, each of us have specific circumstances that cause extreme exhaustion. It's not exactly the same for a gardener, a waiter, a doctor, or a pilot. Even a stay-at-home mom, who many would say doesn't work, can suffer from occupational burnout. Putting too much of yourself into what you do leads to this condition, regardless of your profession and job.

You need to identify what brought you here. Sometimes it's obvious; other times, you need to spend some time in introspection until you discover the exact cause.

What is it about your job that makes you feel anxious or sad or resentful? Maybe your job doesn't bring you fulfillment anymore. Or maybe you still love your job, but:

- You feel underappreciated by your boss or co-workers.
- You have to cooperate with a toxic person who makes you feel terrible.
- You don't know exactly what is expected from you.
- You feel you have no control over your life—other people decide on everything, from your schedule to your salary, and you feel like a slave.
- You don't have enough free time and your personal life suffers.

Your emotions are pointing out that something is wrong or missing. Follow them instead of ignoring or denying what they're telling you.

If you have a boring job, it's not surprising that you feel unmotivated and drained. Repeating the same dull routine, without having your purpose in sight, is really exhausting.

What do you miss? It might be appreciation, adequate compensation for your effort, more free time, more purpose, authenticity, creativity, and freedom.

Use introspection to get to the root of the problem and find out what about your role is bothering you. If you are not sure, try to keep a stress journal where you write about everything that stresses you out. This way, you'll get a clearer picture of causes and triggers, as well as powerful insights. When you think you've found the source of your burnout, think about possible solutions. Brainstorm ways to eliminate the stressors or manage them in the future.

Once you know where the problem lies, you can find ways to change it. Sometimes it requires drastic measures like quitting your job and changing careers. Other times, it's enough to make certain changes in your mindset, approach to work, and everyday life to bring back that lost balance.

5.   Sleep is your superpower

Once you remove yourself from work for a while, it's time to recharge. Lack of sleep is among the most common causes of high stress levels. It's not always easy to get enough quality rest while you are exhausted and suffering from occupational burnout. You might have trouble falling or staying asleep, or the quality of your sleep is poor. Even if you can afford eight hours of uninterrupted sleep, chances are you feel tired even when you wake up. No matter how long you sleep, it seems it's never enough.

So now it's time to pay attention to basic things such as sleep in order to recover. Honestly, it might seem silly to think that just sleeping well for a night or two can make you feel brand new. But it's crucial for your recovery. Take it seriously and start taking steps towards achieving more effective sleep.

Here is some advice on improving your sleep patterns and the quality of your rest:

<u>Let the office stay where it belongs.</u>

Decide that recovery is your top priority now. There's nothing more important that needs to get done. You deserve to rest. Even the simplest devices need regular rest to recharge. So do you.

Too often we are under pressure to be productive all the time. That's why we often undermine the importance of rest, forgetting that it's a natural part of the process. You can't just use your energy all the time without recharging your batteries. It won't work. Accept the fact that rest is sometimes the most productive activity you can do. Free yourself from the constant pressure to accomplish more and more, maximize your time, and be productive in the usual terms. Start appreciating moments of rest and relaxation—they exist for a reason. The proper amount and quality of rest will directly affect your productivity at work.

Don't let anything interrupt your time to rest. Leave everything else aside. This is not the time for thinking about work or other problems. It's not the time to be productive or to achieve anything.

Make your rest a priority. It can be a short nap during the day or just time reserved for doing nothing. But first of all, your night's sleep needs to be long enough to afford proper rest.

<u>Unplug and avoid screens before bedtime.</u>

Realize that you don't have to (and you shouldn't) be available to everyone all the time. It's perfectly fine to turn off your phone or notifications, and be unavailable when the job calls outside of work hours.

Also, avoid all kinds of screens before bedtime. Their blue light tells your mind it's time to be alert and you will have trouble settling down. Establish a new part of the evening routine that includes turning off laptops, phones, computers, and TVs at least two hours before bed. Don't scroll through social media, don't watch TV shows, or (God forbid) the news.

Keep in mind that everything you do before bed you take with you into sleep. Be mindful when choosing what you read, listen to, or think about before going to bed.

<u>Build a relaxing evening routine.</u>

Our minds love routine. It has a calming effect because it give us a sense of predictability and certainty. Your routine before sleep should include going to bed early at the same time every night and involve some relaxing activities. When you go to bed early, it's valuable for your health. Our brain releases chemicals needed for recovery and maintaining our health in perfect condition. So an hour of sleep before midnight is better than an hour after midnight. When you always go to bed at more or less the same time, you'll train your mind to know when to calm down and relax, more efficiently preparing for sleep.

You will fall asleep faster and easier if you are already relaxed when you go to bed. How can you make this happen? Include some calming activities in your bedtime routine. When you unplug and turn off all of the screens, it's time to enjoy some relaxing entertainment such as reading (choose calming and positive books, avoid disturbing ones), doing light yoga or meditation, taking a bubble bath, drawing, cuddling, or anything else that makes you feel serene and calm, and doesn't include electronics or bright light.

You can also include sipping a warm drink before bed, like herbal tea or warm milk. There are special kinds of tea called sleepytime or bedtime teas that contain ingredients that improve sleep.

Bedtime teas have sedative effects, reducing anxiety and stress. They combine anti-anxiety and relaxing herbal ingredients. You've probably already heard of some of them, such as chamomile, valerian, lavender, lemon balm, spearmint, and catnip in the mint family.

Drinking warm milk is also known to help to sleep. Milk contains tryptophan, which impacts the production of chemicals responsible for the sleep-wake cycle, while calcium can help you stay asleep.

<u>Invest in your rest.</u>

People spend about half of their lives sleeping. If you want the latter half to be the best it can be, you need to take care of the former. If you haven't paid a lot of attention to your sleeping habits, chances are you've never bought a proper mattress and bedding.

Now it's time to prioritize rest, so consider investing in it. Choose a mattress that will give your body adequate support during sleep. It's also essential to have proper pillows and covers. Choose natural materials over synthetic ones.

Dark curtains are also great to have in the bedroom so that you can keep any light out of your space. When sleeping in the dark, our body produces chemicals that won't be produced otherwise. The bedroom should be airy and clutter-free, especially free from electronics and screens.

6.   Food can help you overcome burnout

While focusing only on one area in our lives, such as work, we treat our bodies carelessly, not thinking about our physical needs. Chances are you've been eating a lot of junk food, leftovers, carbs; drinking a lot of sweet beverages, coffee, and so on. You may not have lost weight, you might even have gained or became overweight, but your body is actually starving. It lacks good nutrients and real food. To help it recover from extreme exhaustion, you need to take care of your diet. Clean eating and whole foods are your supporters. Good to know, but where to begin?

If you are used to grabbing anything on the go and not planning your meals in advance, this will be a bigger change because it will require planning, practice, and discipline. No one says it's easy, but it's crucial. Your diet is among the first things to consider and change to help yourself recover.

The time of gulping down anything to fuel your body and take in calories while remaining undernourished is over. Let's break bad habits.

<u>Plan in advance.</u>

While giving a 100% of yourself to your job, you've probably formed a habit of eating fast food on the go without thinking. Now you need to do the opposite—plan your diet in advance. This means shopping regulary for groceries (about once a week), stocking healthy food, and planning your weekly menu.

It requires some time and effort at the outset, but you'll spend far less energy on thinking about what to buy and what to cook each day. Decide what you'll eat for breakfast, lunch, dinner, and snacks for the next seven days. Then, make a grocery list and go shopping.

Make healthy choices and focus only on healthy foods such as vegetables, fruit, fish, red meat, and so on. Later, we'll talk more about which foods to include in your diet.

<u>Eat small meals.</u>

Your body is already tired, so this is not the time for skipping meals or trying out any restrictive diets. Your priority should be to keep sugar levels stable and avoid peaks and drops. Switch out big meals for smaller ones and eat five to six times a day. Don't delay your breakfast, eat before 10:00 a.m., and don't think about intermittent fasting for now.

<u>Avoid caffeine.</u>

Caffeine can be overstimulating, triggering your anxiety or encouraging you to spend energy you already lack. It may also interfere with your sleep, and that's the last thing you need. Sleep and rest are crucial for healing from job burnout, so if coffee affects it, then eliminate it from your daily routine for a while.

<u>Avoid sugar.</u>

This is important advice for everyone. We are so used to sweets that we don't see them as treats anymore. Sugar has become just another unhealthy habit you need to get rid of. When you are in a recovery process, the time couldn't be better. It will do you so much good. Acknowledge that we often reach for sweets when we lack energy, need real nutrients, we're tired, or thirsty. You might need a glass of water, a nap, or real food. When you become aware of this, you'll listen to your body and better understand its needs. No, you don't need a bar of chocolate. You might need to tackle some emotional issues. Or you are bored. Or you simply need more water or more sleep.

When you feel the urge to eat something sweet, stop for a moment and ask yourself what you really need. You'll be surprised to discover how often a glass of lemon water or taking a 15 minute nap can cure your craving for sugar. Day by day, nap by nap, and glass by glass, you'll manage to break this bad habit. You'll feel so energized that you'll thank yourself for giving up on your toxic relationship with sugar.

<u>Say no to processed foods.</u>

When we are too busy and exhausted, we reach for quick solutions and that's the worst possible option when it comes to food. Highly processed food is packed in layers of plastic, with a lot of sugar and salt.

The best way to nourish your body properly is to cook your meals yourself. Choose whole foods, fruits and veggies, organic fish and meat, eggs, and seeds to supply the nutrients your body is begging for. You'll feel the difference almost immediately.

Check your food intolerance.

Many people are intolerant to certain foods, such as gluten or dairy. It can provoke different issues, including intestinal problems and mood changes. You might be intolerant to some foods without knowing it. This is why it's recommended to do a blood test for food intolerances.

Eat healthy fats.

We all know that the human brain is made of a huge percentage of fats. But do you eat enough healthy fats in your food? Omega-3 fatty acids are known to increase mood and decrease depression and anxiety symptoms. Healthy fats keep our sugar levels stable and help our body absorb vitamins and antioxidants. It's obvious how they help in beating burnout. Try to include healthy fats in your diet with every meal and don't forget to eat fatty fish at least three times a week.

Using supplements: yes or no?

There's no such thing as a replacement for rest or a healthy diet. There's no magic cure to heal you from burnout. But taking additional vitamins, minerals, and other nutrients through supplements can support and speed up your recovery. To start noticing the effects, reinforce your diet by taking daily supplements for at least 4-6 weeks. Here are a few recommendations:

- Omega 3 + DHA
- Zinc
- B vitamin complex
- Magnesium bisglycinate (450-600 mg per day)
- Liposomal vitamin C
- Ashwagandha
- Holy basil tincture
- High-quality organic green powder
- Flaxseed oil
- Liposomal glutathione
- Caffeine-free electrolyte tablets
- Licorice root extract

7.   Move your body

In times when we are extremely busy, we often neglect to exercise, forgetting that our body is our temple and it should serve us for as long as we live.

When you are too consumed by your work, you let life pass you by. It's time to bring it back, including taking care of your body. It needs movement as much as food or sleep.

Regular exercise affects health in many positive ways. To mention just a few—it reduces stress, blood pressure, and sugar levels; it boosts immunity and improves the release of good chemicals in the brain.

Including a workout in your daily routine will help you a lot in overcoming occupational burnout as well as reduce the consequences of neglecting your body while being super busy.

You already lack energy, I know. It might seem hard to even get out of bed. And I can't blame you if you don't feel like going to the gym and exhausting yourself even more.

A cardio workout is not a good choice right now. Such intense workouts can trigger fight-or-flight mode, provoke cortisol release, and even cause weight gain.

Moderation is the keyword here. You should not push anything too hard—that would only add to your burnout. But an intense workout is not the only way to be active. There are plenty of ways to move your body gently and in ways that can lift your mood.

Think about walking, swimming, yoga, cycling, or some other activity that used to bring you joy. Whatever type of physical activity you choose, be careful not to overexert yourself. If you feel too tired the day after exercising, it might mean that you've been pushing too hard.

Walking

Walking is a natural activity and a gentle way of exercising. Regularly going for a walk will help you relax, decompress, and shape your body while enjoying time in nature. You can reserve that time for walking a dog in the nearest park or hiking in a forest, listening to a podcast while walking along the shore, or whatever suits you. The point is, walking is an easy and natural way of moving that will bring you all the benefits you need from a workout: boosted metabolism, toned body, and a clear mind—all without pushing too hard.

Swimming

If you like swimming, it's also an activity you can use to relax and recharge while exercising. Swimming activates all the muscles, tones the body, and combines workout with the soothing effects of water. It's like exercising, having a massage, and gazing at water at the same time.

Yoga

Yoga might be the most efficient way of working out while you're experiencing occupational burnout. Using a holistic approach, yoga is a workout for your mind, not only your body. Practicing yoga, you'll get a more balanced and toned body, but also clarity of thought and inner peace. It is a perfect choice for recovery because it's gentle yet powerful. It has the capacity to draw your focus inside yourself, helping you come to valuable insights and unblock stagnant energy within your body and mind.

According to yoga philosophy, being out of balance means that your energy centers and channels are not adequately stimulated. Practicing yoga will resolve this and bring your life force back into balance.

Practicing yoga will teach you how to be self-aware. Once you learn that, you'll gain more insight and awareness about everything around you. No more confusion, no more wandering. You'll be aware of how you feel and what exactly causes you to feel that way so you can make needed adjustments and change anything that doesn't serve your highest good. No longer will your job or anything else be more important than you. You'll know exactly what is in alignment with your needs and what doesn't support them. When you go back to work, you'll be revitalized, but now aware of your energy. You'll never again let anything drain it.

You don't need any special expensive equipment for yoga. A mat and comfy clothes are enough. But if you have no experience with this practice, it would be best to find an instructor or a group and take classes. There are plenty of books and videos you can follow to learn yoga, but nothing can compare to real classes with an instructor who will teach you well. Later, when you gain some experience, you can try to do it on your own if you like.

8.   Practice mindfulness

You've probably heard of mindfulness. It's something everybody talks about these days. But did you know it can help you a lot in healing from exhaustion and job burnout? Let's take a look at what mindfulness is.

It's a technique that helps you to be aware and consciously present. Only if you manage to be focused on the here and now, and aware of everything that's going on within you and around you, can you say you're absolutely present. That's what you can achieve through mindfulness. What usually prevents us from being present is the noise in our minds. Through the practice of mindfulness, we can quiet our minds and find stillness and peace so we can become totally aware of the present moment.

In your case, mindfulness will teach you many things:

1. There is so much more to life than your job.
2. Your job doesn't define you. It's not who you are, it's just what you do for a living.
3. There's a higher intelligence within you. You are not your thoughts or actions. If you calm your mind, you'll discover you are much more than this.
4. You can consciously decide what to think, feel, and how to act. You don't have to react to everything around you.
5. You are in control of your focus.
6. You can always find a place of peace and serenity—it's always within you.

Mindfulness will help you reverse the process of exhaustion, recover, and heal. It will teach you how to press pause, save your energy, and never experience occupational burnout again.

9. Mindful breathing

This is the simplest thing you can possibly do: breathe and be aware of doing it. But it is among the most potent mindfulness techniques that can benefit you. Mindful breathing will help you reconnect with yourself, stay grounded, find inner peace, and achieve calm.

How often do you pay attention to your breathing? Most of us are not used to doing it. Do it now. Notice your breathing. Don't try to control or change it; just notice the rhythm and feel the air going in and out of your body.

Focus on movements in your body connected to breathing. Is your breathing deep or shallow?

Place one hand on your stomach and the other one on your chest. Notice which one is moving up and down. If it's the one on your stomach, you do breathe deeply and that's good.

Proper breathing is deep when the air fills your stomach. Most of us breathe shallowly, filling only our chest, which tells our mind that we are in danger. It makes us stressed without us even noticing it.

On the other hand, when you breathe deeply and slowly you send signals that everything's fine, calming yourself.

Relearning how to breathe deeply will help you feel reenergized, feel calm, and find your balance. Once you adopt a new way of breathing, you'll never again allow yourself to forget it and live on a minimum of air. Mindful breathing is intentional and tranquil breathing where you are aware of each moment, of the way the air is moving through your body, and all the sensations it provokes.

You already have everything you need for this mindful activity, but it will require some practice. Day by day it will become your new habit and you'll find yourself more and more aware of your breath. To begin, try to do mindful breathing exercises for five minutes, three times a day.

How do you breathe mindfully?

Sit or lie down in a comfortable position. Choose a time in the day when you know you won't be disturbed for the next ten minutes. Make sure your clothes are comfy.

Take a breath. Feel the air entering your nostrils. Feel its coolness as it goes through your nose. Try to feel it as it fills your lungs and focus on the movement as it expands your belly. Then consciously breathe out, feeling your stomach shrink and the air leaving your lungs. Feel the warm air going out of your body through your nose or mouth. Focus on each tiny sensation during its way in and out. Be aware of every moment of your breath. Focus all of your attention only on that.

You might find it surprising how much goes on in our body while we're merely breathing. It might seem as if there's nothing happening, yet so much is happening all the time. By focusing only on your breath and all the sensations and movement connected to it for as briefly as five minutes at a time, you will feel refreshed, calm, and centered. Just imagine how much more good it will do you when you practice this for longer periods of time and more often.

You can relax, boost your energy, clear your mind, and enhance concentration by simply focusing on your breathing. Doing this every day will tremendously help you regain your balance and recover from occupational burnout in the longterm.

Once you know and appreciate this technique, you'll never lose yourself to burnout again.

10. Mindfulness meditation

As I've said before, being mindful means being consciously present and aware of everything around you and within you. It's impossible to be present and aware if a million thoughts are running through your head all the time.

The most powerful way to calm your mind and become consciously aware is meditation. While going through the burnout phase of your life, this may be the most healing thing you can do for yourself.

Practicing mindfulness meditation will bring you many benefits: stress release, recovery from exhaustion, a sense of ease and flow, reconnection with your body and its sensations, a calm mind, and a state of being present in the here and now.

That's wonderful; let's begin, I hear you saying.

In comencing the practice of mindfulness meditation, there are a few ways to do it and there's not only one right way. The main goal is to relax your body, empty your mind, and focus on the moment and your sensations.

I'll describe the most complete version of mindfulness meditation you can practice. Keep in mind that you can do shorter versions by focusing only on your breath or specific sensations for as briefly as five minutes. This can mean gazing at a candle flame or something like that. The point is in being consciously present and completely aware, no matter how much time you spend.

To begin, find a quiet, comfortable place and choose a time when you know you won't be disturbed for the next 30 minutes.

Make yourself comfortable in a sitting or a supine position. I recommend lying on your back, with your legs straight and your hands beside you, with your palms open to the ceiling.

Take a nice, deep breath. Breathe out. Observe your breathing. Try to notice everything about it—feel the air entering your nostrils. Feel it all the way down in your chest and belly. Feel the movement as your stomach expands and shrinks as the air leaves you. Don't try to control your breathing rhythm; just observe it. Notice every detail and be aware of each moment.

Pay attention to your toes. Be aware of your toes and feet, of the sensations you feel in them. Don't be surprised if you suddenly feel tingling or warmth in your feet. Consciously move your toes and feet a little, be aware of the movement.

Bring your awareness up to your lower legs. Feel the surface beneath them. This kind of focusing on certain parts of the body means you are already relaxing them. Move your focus upward, become aware of your knees, thighs, hips, glutes, and pelvic area. Acknowledge any sensations there.

Move your fingers and feel their movement. Bring awareness to your hands and palms, then

upward to your wrists, lower arms, elbows, and upper arms. Acknowledge all of the sensation in those areas.

Bring your focus to your stomach. Notice how it's moving up and down as you breathe in and out.

Expand it fully, then squeeze abdominals on the exhale.

Fill your chest with the next inhale. Breathe out, allow it to relax. Feel the air filling it and leaving. Feel your muscles moving. Feel the relaxation and calmness.

Bring your awareness to your back now. Try to feel it completely, muscle by muscle, from the lowest to the highest point. Feel the surface under your back. Give your undivided attention to your back, acknowledging all sensation there. This way, you'll relax the entire area. It will feel like receiving a massage from your awareness.

With the next deep breath, become aware of your shoulders. Acknowledge any tension you've been holding there. Just by becoming aware of the tension in your shoulders, you'll be able to relax and release that heavy weight. Feel your muscles relax and loosen.

Bring your focus to your neck and throat. Feel the sensations in those areas—any tension, tingling, warmth; anything you can feel, pleasant or unpleasant. Bring awareness to your head, scalp, forehead, and face. Acknowledge your mouth and tongue, your eyes, and any sensation on your face.

Once you have entirely scanned you body with your undivided attention, it's finally relaxed in a completely new way from head to toe. You're aware of all of your muscles and your breathing.

Now bring your attention to your skin. Feel the surface of your body. Feel what is beneath your body. Notice the touch of fabric, your clothes, sheets, covers, anything that touches your body. Feel the textures.

Notice the temperature of the air around you and the temperature on the surface of your skin. Feel your inner warmth, become aware of it.

Notice if you can smell anything. Don't try to define it, name it, or judge it; just feel and acknowledge what your senses have to tell you.

Pay attention to sounds. What can you hear? It might be the wind, rain, birds singing, dogs barking, voices from outside, traffic, sounds from next door, sounds of home appliances—whatever you can hear. Again, try not to name them or think about them. Just focus on sound, on the vibration of the air sensed by your ears.

Sometimes it can be enough just to close your eyes and focus completely on the sounds around you. Or you can burn a candle and watch it for a while. Whenever you feel the need to ground yourself and de-stress, press pause, and focus on your senses, five minutes sometimes can be all that you need to regain your balance. This can be especially useful once you go back to work. Every time you feel you are losing your inner peace, bring yourself back to the present moment using mindfulness techniques.

11. Awareness

Meditation and breathing exercises are not the only ways to practice mindfulness and be aware. You can do it whenever you want during whatever activity. Just remind yourself to bring your attention back to the present moment. Notice what you can feel with your senses. Ground yourself in the here and now, and be consciously aware of the moment. Some of the best opportunities to practice mindfulness are usual activities that don't require your special attention and effort, like going for a walk, taking a shower, cooking, cleaning, and eating.

For instance, when you're in the shower focus on the touch of the water droplets on your skin, listen to the sound of the shower, feel the touch of your hands, smell the scents of your shower gel or soap. Feel the temperature of the water and the air around you. Focus only on the part of the body you're showering at the moment, until your whole body is clean. You'll be surprised by how refreshed you feel. You won't need to go to a spa—you'll feel like you're experiencing one at home, in your own bathroom. That's the difference awareness makes.

You can practice mindfulness while taking a walk, for example. Be aware of each move your legs make. Focus on your breathing and be aware of each moment, every breath in and out. Notice the sights, sounds, colors, smells, the world around you. Can you imagine how much there is to be aware of? Mindful walking is completely different from taking a walk totally occupied by your thoughts, hardly noticing anything around you. And it's a shame because by being too much in your head, you are missing out on your only life.

Ordinary, everyday jobs don't have to be chores. If you decide to tackle them completely aware and mindful, cooking a meal or cleaning the kitchen can be a relaxing experience. Just focus on the smells, textures, colors, touch, movement, and breathing. There's not even one single moment in the day that can't be fabulous if you live it in complete awareness.

All of that will significantly improve the quality of your life and reduce your levels of stress. It's unnecessary to highlight how important this is while you are recovering from burnout. But when you also start applying your new mindfulness skills at work, you'll notice big changes. You'll be more focused on the work in front of you than on the negativity that bothers you. You'll pay more attention to enjoying the process than merely on the final goal. You'll be calmer and less prone to exhaustion.

12. Boost your social life

Since we are human beings, we crave social connections to stay healthy and happy. While you are giving your best at work, you might neglect your personal relationships. While you're entirely consumed by your job, people who love you get very little of your time and attention.

While healing from occupational burnout, it's time to heal your relationships too. The job is not the one who will be there for you to love you, support you, and offer you comfort and emotional connection. Nothing in life matters more than your loved ones. That's why you need to boost your personal and social life, creating a balance between it and your work. Spending time with family and friends makes you feel loved and cared for, reminding you that your job is not your whole life or the most important thing in the world.

It's hard to make time in your busy schedule for friends and family while you are obsessed with work. It's even harder to reach out to people when you feel drained and exhausted. But it's a must. Even if you don't feel like it, reach out to people you know that care for you. They will be pleased to help.

Talk to a trusted friend or family member. Tell them what you're going through. You might be surprised to discover how much support and understanding you can get when you open up a bit and speak sincerely.

Engage in family gatherings and go out with friends. It doesn't have to be a night out if you don't feel like it. It might be just a walk, hanging out together, going for a drink, or sipping coffee.

There are many ways to connect with people. You can play with kids if you have your own or with those of friends and family. Offer support and help to those who might need it. Volunteer or engage in group activities. You can connect with people who have the same interests as you, knowing that you're engaging in a good cause and involved in something bigger than yourself.

Positive social connections are the key to a long and fulfilling life. Cultivate and maintain them. If you haven't done it in a while, they need some special care now. But it will all pay off in stronger bonds, better connections, more fulfillment, and joy. Happiness grows when it's shared with others.

13. Do more of what makes you happy

Can you even remember what used to make you happy? What you loved to do as a child or before you started to be overwhelmed by your job? Do you know the activity that made you forget about time and space? It might be anything from drawing, painting, dancing, singing, gardening, reading, to anything in the world. It might be clay modeling, scrapbooking, knitting, yoga, playing golf, spending time in nature. No matter what you choose, the goal is to feel alive, joyful, and cheerful.

Kids know how to do things with their whole being. They choose activities that make them happy and then give them their undivided attention, without thinking about time or other unimportant things. Most of us have lost that inner child and the ability to play as life moves on. Instead, we are taught to be serious all the time, to be always busy, productive, and committed to what we are supposed to do.

Free time and joyful activities are something we must deserve by working hard and giving up any satisfaction in the meantime. But you can't expect to have a happy, balanced life when you lack joy, laughter, and play.

It's time to include these activities in your everyday life. If you can remember what you loved in the past, that's a great place to start. If comedies made you laugh out loud, it's time to start watching them again. Find your favorite movies or TV shows, make some popcorn, and enjoy them. If you loved reading funny books, don't hesitate to track them down. Did you love to spend time in nature? Go to the park, the nearest forest, a lake, a mountain, a river, a beach—be outside as much as you like. Loved crafting? Find some supplies and get to work.

If you don't know what makes you feel good, it's time to find out. Attempt different activities and see how you feel. You can try out ones that require company, such as sports activities. View different kinds of art, consume different genres of books and movies, attend different events, and take stock of your mood and emotions. That's the guiding system you need to learn to trust.

Once you discover what makes you happy, make space for it in your schedule. If you don'tt, you'll never make time for it. No matter if it's reading, yoga classes, visiting museums, or singing in a church, you need to make time for it among your priorities. As the saying goes, you can't pour from an empty cup. Nourish your soul first. That's where it all comes from. A nourished soul will help you regain your balance and never let you fall into burnout again.

14. Rearrange your priorities

We all have the same 24 hours each day. The difference is in the way we choose to spend them. "I have no time for..." is not the truth. It just means, "It's not a priority." And that's perfectly fine. But. What *is* a priority?

Suffering from occupational burnout is a sure sign that your priorities are out of balance. You've allowed your job to become the only priority, and all other areas of your life suffer because it consumes all of your time and energy.

If your number one priority is your work, it's not healthy. We all need at least several areas to function well in our lives in order to experience balance and prosperity. There should be your health (physical and mental), family, friends, relationships, self-growth, service to society or a meaningful cause, spirituality, free time, and exercise. Consider each of them. For harmony, you need all the parts to work well.

Do you have a clear vision for your life? Where you want to go and why? If you do, remember it and remember why you started to do what you do in the first place. What were your motivations and your goals? Do they fit in your present life? Do they refer to you as the person you are now?

If they don't or if you've never created a clear vision for yourself, it's time to do it now. Imagine your dream life. What would you like to do? How much money do you want to have? Who do you want to live with? How do you want to feel?

If your health is a top priority, isn't it silly to sacrifice it for work, for a paid bonus, or anyone else's recognition? If health is the priority, don't eat junk food.

When it's about work, what is the job you'd do if you didn't have to earn a living? Yes, if money wasn't an issue, what would you do?

Now, think if you could fit it into reality somehow. Maybe you don't want to change your career and become an artist, for example, but you could bring some creativity into your work.

What else could you change? If you have problems in personal relationships with co-workers, you might want to seek solutions, work on your communication skills, or change jobs. If a lack of control is what bothers you the most, maybe you would feel better as an entrepreneur.

Make needed adjustments in your life and career to make it as close as it can be to your vision, following your priorities.

When you have a strong "why," balanced priorities, and you live according to your values, you are not prone to exhaustion or burnout in any field in the future.

How to Prevent Occupational Burnout in the Future

As the saying goes, change the situation. If you can't change the situation, change yourself.

It's true in this case, too. If you can, change what's bothering you. It might be your job, co-workers, and place in the organization. If you can't gain control over those things or don't want to change them, you need to change something within you: your beliefs, perspective, focus, attitude, or mindset. In either case, don't allow the same things to bring you to exhaustion again.

Everything we've talked about here will help you overcome burnout and regain your balance. But you should incorporate them into your daily life to prevent it from happening again. In other words, you need to live a balanced and healthy life with all aspects active, ensuring that your goals are in alignment with your values. When you build a healthy foundation, no stress can make you burn out and you won't allow your job to become the only thing you live for.

In short, you need to take care of your life as a whole, not as a time to work. Take care of your body, mind, and spirit; grow your relationships, feed your soul, and work for a living—not the other way around.

Decide on your priorities.

When you know the place of everything on your list of priorities, you always know what's more important than something else, and it's easy to choose where to direct your energy and time. Your work can't be the only thing that matters in your life. And it must not cost you health, relationships, or happiness.

Don't neglect your vision.

When you have a vision of your perfect life, you have a north star. You can pause any time and ask yourself, *Does this bring me closer to my dream life or pull me further away from it?* This way, you'll always know exactly what to do. If those extra hours at work really bring you closer, you'll be able to tackle them without exhaustion. But if they mean sacrificing your health or missing your kid's school play—that's not even close to your dream life.

Treat your body with love and appreciation.

Your body is your temple. Show it respect and gratitude. No one who loves their body will force it to sit in front of a computer all day long. Don't malnourish your body, fuel it with junk, or starve it.

Don't force it to stay awake in the name of work. Don't allow stress to overwhelm you.

Slow down. Breathe. Be mindful. Rest as much as you need. Nourish your body with healthy food. Hydrate it well. Your brain is made of a lot of water. When you are hydrated, your thoughts are clean. Stretch your body, exercise regularly, take walks. There's no price for effort. No one will reward you for pushing yourself hard and punishing your body—for what? Take care of yourself and the only body you have.

<u>Take care of your mind.</u>

Mental hygiene is a must and everybody needs to practice it if they want to be happy. Being conscious and aware of your thoughts and emotions is the first step towards mental balance and inner peace. All of the changes you want to experience in the material world begin in your mind. That's why it's crucial to reexamine your beliefs, learn how to control your thoughts, and manage your emotions. This way you become the master of your mind and your life, instead of coasting randomly on autopilot.

There are numerous ways to practice mental hygiene. You can start with books on the subject, videos, podcasts, yoga, meditation, or self-development techniques and tools.

<u>Get off the hamster wheel.</u>

Focusing too much on work might feel like being in a hamster's spinning wheel or engaging in a rat race. Press pause. Get off the wheel. Take a deep breath and relax. You don't have to feel stressed all the time. You don't have to be busy all the time. You don't have to rush.

Take a break. Rest and recharge. Then, rearrange your life. Ask yourself what you truly desire and what your soul craves. Spend some time in silence, in nature, in introspection. We all need space to process things and we often lack it because we have no time. Give yourself permission to take as much time as you need, see things for what they truly are, and be honest with yourself.

Let go of all the "musts" and "have tos." The world won't stop spinning. Nothing terrible will happen. Slow down, feel the life around you and within you, and appreciate it. When you feel rested and reenergized, take back your power, take your life in your hands, and decide on every single thing about it—including your job, your priorities, your big and small dreams, and every moment of your days. Listen to your emotions and let your soul guide you to the places and activities that feel like home.